30 YOGA STRETCHES FOR THE OFFICE WORKERS

BY

RIZWAN CHUHAN

3

Table of Contents

6

7

INTRODUCTION

In today's world, many people spend a significant amount of time sitting in front of a computer or desk for work. This sedentary lifestyle can lead to a variety of health issues, including poor posture, muscle tension, and chronic pain. Yoga stretching has become an increasingly popular way for office workers to counteract these negative effects and improve their overall physical and mental wellbeing.

8

This book, "30 Yoga Stretches for the Office Workers," is designed to provide practical guidance for office workers who want to incorporate yoga stretching into their daily routine. It includes a variety of stretches specifically targeted to address common areas of tension in the neck, shoulders, back, hips, wrists, and hands. Additionally, the book includes tips for safe stretching, explanations of basic yoga principles, and three different yoga routines to fit into any office worker's busy schedule.

By incorporating these yoga stretches into their daily routine, office workers can improve their posture, reduce muscle tension, increase flexibility, and promote relaxation. This book aims to provide a practical guide to help office workers achieve these benefits and improve their overall health and wellbeing.

10

Importance of stretching for office workers

Stretching is an essential part of maintaining good physical health and is particularly important for office workers who spend prolonged periods sitting at a desk. Sitting for extended periods can cause muscles to become tight and tense, leading to pain and discomfort in the neck, shoulders, back, hips, and legs.

Stretching helps to counteract these negative effects by improving circulation, increasing range of motion, and reducing muscle tension. Stretching also helps to improve posture, which is important for office workers who spend long hours sitting in front of a computer. Poor posture can lead to a variety of health issues, including neck pain, back pain, headaches, and fatigue.

In addition to physical benefits, stretching also has mental and emotional benefits. Stretching can help to reduce stress, promote relaxation, and improve overall mood. For office workers who may experience high levels of stress on a daily basis, stretching can be an effective tool for managing stress and improving mental wellbeing.

Overall, stretching is a simple yet effective way for office workers to maintain good physical health, reduce the risk of injury, and improve mental and emotional wellbeing. Incorporating regular stretching into a daily routine can have significant long-term benefits for office workers.

13

Benefits of yoga stretches

Yoga stretches offer a multitude of benefits for the mind and body, making it an ideal practice for office workers looking to improve their overall health and wellbeing. Some of the key benefits of yoga stretches include:

Increased flexibility: Yoga stretches focus on lengthening and loosening the muscles, which can improve flexibility and range of motion.

Reduced muscle tension: Yoga stretches help to release muscle tension, which can alleviate pain and discomfort in the neck, shoulders, back, hips, and legs.

Improved posture: Many yoga stretches help to strengthen the muscles that support good posture, which can reduce the risk of developing posture-related health issues such as neck pain, back pain, and headaches.

Enhanced relaxation: Yoga stretches incorporate breathing techniques and mindful movements, which can promote relaxation and reduce stress.

Improved balance and coordination: Many yoga stretches require balance and coordination, which can improve overall physical stability and reduce the risk of falls or other injuries.

Improved mental wellbeing: Yoga stretches can also improve mental wellbeing by reducing stress and promoting relaxation, which can improve overall mood and emotional health.

Overall, yoga stretches offer a wide range of benefits for both the mind and body, making it an ideal practice for office workers looking to improve their overall health and wellbeing.

17

Purpose of the book

The purpose of "30 Yoga Stretches for the Office Workers" is to provide a practical guide for office workers who want to incorporate yoga stretching into their daily routine. The book is designed to be accessible to individuals of all levels of experience, from those who have never practiced yoga before to those who are experienced yogis.

The book includes a variety of yoga stretches specifically targeted to address common areas of tension in the neck, shoulders, back, hips, wrists, and hands. The stretches are easy to follow and can be done in a small space, making them ideal for office workers who may not have access to a yoga studio or other large workout space.

In addition to the stretches themselves, the book also includes tips for safe stretching, explanations of basic yoga principles, and three different yoga routines to fit into any office worker's busy schedule. By incorporating these stretches and routines into their daily routine, office workers can improve their posture, reduce muscle tension, increase flexibility, and promote relaxation.

The ultimate goal of this book is to provide office workers with the tools they need to maintain good physical and mental health despite the demands of their job. By practicing yoga stretches regularly, office workers can improve their overall health and wellbeing and lead a more balanced, fulfilling life.

Basic principles of yoga stretching

Yoga stretching is a practice that is grounded in several basic principles. These principles guide the practice and help to ensure that individuals are practicing safely and effectively. Some of the basic principles of yoga stretching include:

Mind-body connection: Yoga stretching emphasizes the connection between the mind and body. Practitioners are encouraged to focus on their breath and to pay attention to the sensations in their body as they move through the stretches.

Awareness: Yoga stretching also emphasizes awareness of the present moment. Practitioners are encouraged to focus on the present and to let go of any thoughts or worries about the past or future.

Alignment: Proper alignment is essential for safe and effective yoga stretching. Practitioners are encouraged to maintain proper alignment throughout each stretch, which can help to prevent injury and promote optimal benefits.

Breath: Breath is an essential aspect of yoga stretching. Practitioners are encouraged to breathe deeply and rhythmically, which can help to reduce stress, promote relaxation, and increase oxygen flow to the muscles.

Patience and consistency: Yoga stretching is a practice that requires patience and consistency. Practitioners are encouraged to be patient with themselves and to practice regularly in order to achieve optimal benefits.

By following these basic principles, individuals can practice yoga stretching safely and effectively, and experience the many benefits that this practice has to offer.

24

Explanation of yoga stretching

Yoga stretching is a type of physical exercise that involves holding different poses or postures while focusing on breath and body awareness. The goal of yoga stretching is to improve flexibility, strength, balance, and mental clarity.

Yoga stretching is typically practiced on a yoga mat or other soft surface, and can be done in a variety of settings, from yoga studios to the comfort of one's own home. During a yoga stretching session, practitioners will move through a series of poses, each held for several breaths or longer.

Yoga stretching poses are designed to stretch and strengthen different muscles and parts of the body, such as the hamstrings, hips, back, and shoulders. Many yoga stretching poses also involve twisting or bending the spine, which can improve overall spinal health and flexibility.

One of the unique aspects of yoga stretching is its emphasis on breath and mindfulness. Practitioners are encouraged to focus on their breath and to move mindfully through each pose, paying attention to the sensations in their body and letting go of any distracting thoughts.

Yoga stretching can be beneficial for people of all ages and fitness levels, as the poses can be modified to suit individual needs and abilities. Regular practice of yoga stretching can help to improve overall physical health, reduce stress and anxiety, and promote mental clarity and wellbeing.

27

Importance of breathing during stretching

Breathing is a crucial component of yoga stretching, as it helps to facilitate the movement of the body, regulate the nervous system, and promote relaxation. There are several reasons why breathing is important during stretching:

Oxygenation: During yoga stretching, the body requires an increased supply of oxygen to the muscles in order to maintain the stretches. Deep, rhythmic breathing helps to increase oxygenation to the muscles, which can improve overall physical performance and prevent muscle cramping or injury.

Stress reduction: Deep breathing can help to reduce stress and anxiety, which can be especially beneficial during stretching. When we hold a stretch, it can be easy to tense up and hold our breath, but deep breathing helps to keep the body relaxed and calm.

Mind-body connection: Breathing is an important aspect of the mind-body connection that is emphasized in yoga stretching. By focusing on the breath and coordinating it with the movement of the body, practitioners can cultivate a greater awareness of their physical and mental state.

Relaxation: Focusing on the breath during yoga stretching can also promote relaxation and reduce tension in the body. By consciously slowing down the breath and taking deep, full breaths, practitioners can promote a state of relaxation that can be beneficial for both physical and mental health.

Overall, breathing is an essential aspect of yoga stretching, as it helps to regulate the body's response to stress, improve physical performance, and promote relaxation and mental clarity. By focusing on the breath during yoga stretching, practitioners can enhance the benefits of the practice and cultivate a greater sense of overall wellbeing.

31

Safety tips

When practicing yoga stretches as an office worker, it is important to keep in mind the following safety tips:

Listen to your body: Pay attention to how your body feels during the stretches, and stop or modify any poses that cause pain or discomfort.

Warm up: Before starting any yoga stretching, it is important to warm up your muscles. Consider doing some light cardio or stretching beforehand to prepare your body for the practice.

Use props: Props such as blocks or straps can help to support your body during stretches and ensure that you are practicing safely and effectively.

Respect your limits: It is important to respect your body's limits and not push yourself too far during stretches. Remember that flexibility takes time to develop and cannot be forced.

Stay hydrated: Drink plenty of water before, during, and after your yoga stretching practice to stay hydrated and avoid dehydration.

Avoid over-stretching: While stretching is important, it is important to avoid over-stretching, which can cause injury. Instead, focus on maintaining proper alignment and holding each stretch for a comfortable amount of time.

Consult a professional: If you have any pre-existing medical conditions or concerns about practicing yoga stretching, it is important to consult with a healthcare professional or a qualified yoga instructor before starting a practice.

By following these safety tips, you can ensure that you are practicing yoga stretching safely and effectively, and minimize the risk of injury or discomfort.

30 Yoga Stretches for office workers

Here are 30 yoga stretches for office workers:

1. Seated Forward Bend

2. Seated Spinal Twist

3. Cat-Cow Stretch

4. Downward-Facing Dog

5. Upward-Facing Dog

6. Child's Pose

7. Cobra Pose

8. Plank Pose

9. Tree Pose

10. Warrior II Pose

11. Triangle Pose

12. Extended Side Angle Pose

13. Half Moon Pose

14. Bound Angle Pose

15. Head-to-Knee Forward Bend

16. Standing Forward Bend

17. Camel Pose

18. Cow Face Pose

19. Pigeon Pose

20. Seated Butterfly Pose

21. Corpse Pose

22. Sun Salutation A

23. Sun Salutation B

24. Standing Half Forward Bend

25. Dolphin Pose

26. Bridge Pose

27.	Fish Pose

28.	Extended Puppy Pose

29.	Shoulder Stand

30.	Fisherman's Pose

These stretches can help to improve flexibility, reduce tension and stress, and promote overall physical and mental wellbeing. It is important to remember to practice these stretches safely and mindfully, following the basic principles of yoga stretching and the safety tips outlined above.

Neck and shoulder stretches

Office workers often experience tension and discomfort in the neck and shoulder areas due to prolonged sitting and computer use. Here are some yoga stretches that can help to relieve tension and improve mobility in the neck and shoulders:

Seated Neck Rolls: Sit comfortably in a chair with your feet flat on the ground. Drop your chin to your chest and slowly roll your head to the right. Hold for a few breaths, then roll your head back to center and repeat on the left side.

Seated Eagle Arms: Sit up straight in your chair and bring your arms out in front of you. Cross your right arm over your left and bring your palms to touch. Lift your elbows up and hold for a few breaths, then release and repeat with the left arm over the right.

Seated Shoulder Shrugs: Sit up straight in your chair and lift your shoulders up towards your ears. Hold for a few breaths, then release and repeat a few times.

Seated Half Cow-Faced Pose: Sit up straight in your chair and bring your left hand behind your back, palm facing out. Bring your right arm up and over your head, bending at the elbow and trying to touch your left hand. Hold for a few breaths, then repeat on the other side.

Seated Thread the Needle: Sit up straight in your chair and bring your right arm up and over your head, bending at the elbow. Reach your left hand underneath your right arm and hold onto your right shoulder blade. Hold for a few breaths, then repeat on the other side.

Seated Neck Stretch: Sit up straight in your chair and interlace your fingers behind your head. Gently pull your head forward and down, tucking your chin to your chest. Hold for a few breaths, then release. Remember to practice these stretches mindfully, paying attention to your body and any sensations you may be experiencing. Avoid any stretches that cause pain or discomfort, and modify them as needed to suit your individual needs and limitations.

42

Neck roll

The neck roll is a simple and effective yoga stretch that can help to relieve tension and improve mobility in the neck and shoulders. Here's how to do it:

1.   Begin by sitting up straight in a comfortable seated position, either on a chair or on the floor.

2.   Take a few deep breaths to relax your body and center your mind.

3.   Drop your chin down towards your chest and slowly begin to roll your head to the right.

4.	Allow your head to continue rolling to the right until your right ear is over your right shoulder.

5.	Hold the stretch for a few breaths, feeling a gentle stretch along the left side of your neck and shoulder.

6.	Slowly begin to roll your head back to center, then continue rolling to the left.

7.	Hold the stretch on the left side for a few breaths, feeling a gentle stretch along the right side of your neck and shoulder.

8.	Roll your head back to center and repeat the sequence a few times, moving slowly and mindfully.

It's important to remember to move slowly and gently during the neck roll, as the neck is a delicate area that can be easily injured if strained or pushed too hard. If you experience any pain or discomfort during the stretch, stop immediately and consult a healthcare professional or qualifi ed yoga instructor for guidance.

45

Shoulder shrugs

Shoulder shrugs are a simple and effective yoga stretch that can help to release tension in the shoulders and improve mobility in the upper back. Here's how to do it:

1.   Begin by sitting up straight in a comfortable seated position, either on a chair or on the floor.

2.   Take a few deep breaths to relax your body and center your mind.

3.   Lift your shoulders up towards your ears, squeezing your shoulder blades together.

4.   Hold the stretch for a few breaths, feeling a gentle stretch and release of tension in your shoulders and upper back.

5.   Slowly release the stretch and let your shoulders drop down and back, feeling a sense of relaxation and release in your upper body.

6.   Repeat the sequence a few times, moving slowly and mindfully. It's important to remember to move slowly and gently during shoulder shrugs, as the shoulders are a sensitive area that can be easily strained or injured if pushed too hard. If you experience any pain or discomfort during the stretch, stop

immediately and consult a healthcare professional or qualified yoga instructor for guidance.

48

Shoulder rolls

Shoulder rolls are a simple and effective yoga stretch that can help to release tension in the shoulders and improve mobility in the upper back. Here's how to do it:

1.   Begin by sitting up straight in a comfortable seated position, either on a chair or on the floor.

2.   Take a few deep breaths to relax your body and center your mind.

3.   Lift your shoulders up towards your ears, squeezing your shoulder blades together.

4.   Slowly roll your shoulders back and down, drawing your shoulder blades towards each other and down your back.

5.   Repeat the sequence a few times, moving slowly and mindfully. As you roll your shoulders, try to visualize the tension and stress in your shoulders melting away and releasing with each movement. You may also want to coordinate your breath with the movement, inhaling as you lift your shoulders up and exhaling as you roll them back and down.

It's important to remember to move slowly and gently during shoulder rolls, as the shoulders are a sensitive area that can be easily strained or injured if pushed too hard. If you experience any pain or discomfort during the stretch, stop immediately and consult a healthcare professional or qualified yoga instructor for guidance.

Shoulder stretch

The shoulder stretch is a yoga posture that can help to release tension and increase flexibility in the shoulders and upper back. Here's how to do it:

1.   Begin by standing up straight with your feet hip-width apart and your arms at your sides.

2.   Take a few deep breaths to relax your body and center your mind.

3.   Bring your left arm across your chest, holding it just below the elbow with your right hand.

4.   Gently pull your left arm towards your body, feeling a stretch in your left shoulder and upper back.

5.   Hold the stretch for a few breaths, feeling the tension release with each exhale.

6.   Release the stretch and repeat on the other side, bringing your right arm across your chest and holding it with your left hand.

7.   Hold the stretch for a few breaths, feeling a gentle stretch and release of tension in your right shoulder and upper back.

8.   Repeat the sequence a few times on each side, moving slowly and mindfully.

As you hold the shoulder stretch, try to maintain a tall and open posture, avoiding the temptation to round your shoulders or collapse your chest. You can also experiment with different hand positions and angles to find the variation of the stretch that feels most effective for your body.

It's important to remember to move slowly and gently during the shoulder stretch, as the shoulders are a sensitive area that can be easily strained or injured if pushed too hard. If you experience any pain or discomfort during the stretch, stop immediately and consult a healthcare professional or qualified yoga instructor for guidance.

Back stretches

Back stretches can help to release tension and increase flexibility in the muscles and joints of the back. Here are a few examples of yoga stretches that can be done to stretch the back:

1.   Cat-cow stretch: Begin on your hands and knees, with your wrists directly under your shoulders and your knees under your hips. Inhale, arch your back and lift your tailbone and head toward the ceiling, creating a curve

in your spine (cow). Exhale, round your spine and tuck your chin toward your chest (cat). Move back and forth between cow and cat for several breaths, keeping your movements smooth and fluid.

2.   Seated forward fold: Sit on the floor with your legs straight out in front of you. Inhale, lengthen your spine and lift your arms overhead. Exhale, fold forward from the hips, reaching for your feet or shins. Keep your spine long and your chest open as you hold the stretch for several breaths.

3.   Child's pose: Begin on your hands and knees, then lower your hips back toward your heels and stretch your arms out in front of you. Rest your forehead on the mat and take several deep breaths, feeling the stretch in your lower back.

4.   Downward-facing dog: Start on your hands and knees, then lift your hips up and back, straightening your arms and legs and forming an inverted V shape with your body. Keep your heels grounded and your head relaxed as you hold the pose for several

breaths, feeling a stretch in your back, hamstrings, and calves.

It's important to remember to move slowly and gently during back stretches, avoiding any sudden or jerky movements that could cause injury. If you experience any pain or discomfort during the stretch, stop immed

59

Cat-Cow stretch

The Cat-Cow stretch is a yoga posture that can help to stretch and release tension in the spine and improve mobility in the back. Here's how to do it:

1.   Begin on your hands and knees, with your wrists directly under your shoulders and your knees under your hips.
2.   Take a few deep breaths to relax your body and center your mind.
3.   Inhale, arch your back and lift your tailbone and head toward the

ceiling, creating a curve in your spine (Cow pose).

4.   Exhale, round your spine and tuck your chin toward your chest, feeling a stretch in your upper back (Cat pose).

5.   Continue to move back and forth between Cow and Cat poses with each inhale and exhale, moving slowly and smoothly.

6.   As you move through the poses, try to focus on creating a fluid, wave-like motion through your spine, moving from the tailbone to the crown of the head.

It's important to remember to move slowly and gently during the Cat-

Cow stretch, avoiding any sudden or jerky movements that could cause injury. You can also experiment with different variations of the stretch, such as holding each pose for longer or adding in subtle movements like circling the hips or shoulders.

If you experience any pain or discomfort during the stretch, stop immediately and consult a healthcare professional or qualified yoga instructor for guidance.

62

Spinal Twist

The spinal twist is a yoga pose that helps to stretch and release tension in the spine, hips, and lower back. Here's how to do it:

1.   Start by sitting on the floor with your legs extended in front of you.

2.   Bend your right knee and bring your right foot to the outside of your left thigh, placing it on the floor.

3.   Take your left arm and bring it across your body, placing your left hand on your right knee.

4.   Inhale and lengthen your spine, sitting up tall.

5.   As you exhale, gently twist your torso to the right, using your left arm to deepen the stretch.

6.   Hold the twist for several breaths, feeling a stretch in your spine and hips.

7.   To come out of the pose, inhale and release the twist, then switch sides and repeat the stretch on the other side.

It's important to move slowly and gently during the spinal twist, avoiding any sudden or jerky movements that could cause injury. If you experience any pain or discomfort during the stretch, stop immediately and consult a healthcare professional or qualified yoga instructor for guidance. You can also modify the stretch as needed, using props like blankets or blocks to help support your body and deepen the stretch.

Forward Fold

The forward fold is a yoga pose that can help to stretch the hamstrings, calves, and lower back, while also calming the mind and relieving stress. Here's how to do it:

1.   Start by standing with your feet hip-width apart, with your arms at your sides.

2.   Inhale and lift your arms up overhead, reaching toward the ceiling.

3.   As you exhale, hinge forward at the hips, keeping your spine

straight and your knees slightly bent.

4.   Allow your hands to rest on your thighs, shins, or the floor, depending on your flexibility.

5.   Relax your neck and shoulders, and let your head hang down toward the floor.

6.   Take several deep breaths in this pose, feeling a stretch in your hamstrings and lower back.

7.   To come out of the pose, slowly roll up to a standing position, vertebra by vertebra, with your head coming up last.

It's important to remember to move slowly and gently during the forward fold, avoiding any sudden or jerky movements that could cause injury. You can also modify the stretch as needed, using props like a block or strap to help support your body and deepen the stretch. If you experience any pain or discomfort during the stretch, stop immediately and consult a healthcare professional or qualified yoga instructor for guidance.

Cobra pose

The Cobra pose is a yoga posture that can help to strengthen the back muscles and improve posture, while also stretching the chest and shoulders. Here's how to do it:

Begin by lying face down on your mat, with your legs extended behind you and your hands placed on the floor under your shoulders.

Press your hands into the mat, keeping your elbows close to your body.

Inhale and lift your chest off the mat, using your back muscles to lift yourself up.

Keep your gaze forward and your neck in a neutral position.

Hold the pose for a few breaths, feeling a stretch in your chest and shoulders.

To come out of the pose, exhale and slowly lower your chest back down to the mat.

It's important to move slowly and gently during the Cobra pose, avoiding any sudden or jerky movements that could cause injury. You can also modify the stretch as needed, using props like a block or blanket to help support your body and deepen the stretch. If you experience any pain or discomfort during the stretch, stop immediately and consult a healthcare professional or qualified yoga instructor for guidance.

71

Leg and hip stretches

Sure, here are three leg and hip stretches for office workers:

Pigeon Pose: Start on all fours with your hands and knees on the mat. Bring your right knee forward, placing it behind your right wrist. Extend your left leg behind you, keeping your hips square. Slowly lower your body down to the mat and rest your forehead on your hands or on a block. Hold for a few breaths, then repeat on the other side.

Seated Forward Bend: Sit on the mat with your legs extended in front of you. Inhale and lengthen your spine, then exhale and fold forward, reaching for your feet or ankles. If you can't reach your feet, use a strap or towel to gently pull yourself forward. Hold for a few breaths, then slowly release the pose.

Butterfly Pose: Sit on the mat with the soles of your feet together, allowing your knees to fall open to the sides. Inhale and lengthen your spine, then exhale and fold forward, allowing your forehead to rest on the mat or on a block. You can use your elbows to gently press down on your thighs, deepening the stretch in your hips. Hold for a few breaths, then release the pose.

Remember to move slowly and gently during these stretches, and to breathe deeply throughout each pose. If you experience any pain or discomfort, stop immediately and consult a healthcare professional or qualified yoga instructor for guidance.

74

Seated Forward Bend

Seated Forward Bend is a yoga posture that can help to stretch the hamstrings, lower back, and hips. It's a great stretch for office workers who spend a lot of time sitting at a desk. Here's how to do it:

Start by sitting on the floor with your legs extended in front of you.

Inhale and lift your arms up overhead, reaching toward the ceiling.

As you exhale, hinge forward at the hips, keeping your spine straight and your knees slightly bent.

Allow your hands to rest on your thighs, shins, or the floor, depending on your flexibility.

Relax your neck and shoulders, and let your head hang down toward your knees.

Take several deep breaths in this pose, feeling a stretch in your hamstrings and lower back.

To come out of the pose, inhale and slowly lift your torso back up to a seated position.

It's important to remember to move slowly and gently during the Seated Forward Bend, avoiding any sudden or jerky movements that could cause injury. You can also modify the stretch as needed, using props like a strap or block to help support your body and deepen the stretch. If you experience any pain or discomfort during the stretch, stop immediately and consult a healthcare professional or qualified yoga instructor for guidance.

Butterfly stretch

The Butterfly stretch, also known as the Bound Angle Pose, is a yoga posture that can help to stretch the inner thighs, groin, and hips. Here's how to do it:

Start by sitting on the floor with your legs extended in front of you.

Bend your knees and bring the soles of your feet together, allowing your knees to fall open to the sides.

Use your hands to gently grasp your feet or ankles, pulling your heels in toward your body.

Sit up tall, lengthening your spine and drawing your shoulder blades down and back.

Take several deep breaths in this pose, feeling a stretch in your inner thighs and groin.

To deepen the stretch, you can gently press down on your thighs with your elbows, encouraging your knees to move closer to the floor.

To come out of the pose, release your feet and extend your legs in front of you.

Remember to move slowly and gently during the Butterfly stretch, and to breathe deeply throughout each pose. If you experience any pain or discomfort, stop immediately and consult a healthcare professional or qualified yoga instructor for guidance. You can also modify the stretch as needed, using props like a block or blanket to help support your body and deepen the stretch.

Figure four stretch

The Figure Four stretch, also known as the Pigeon Pose, is a yoga posture that can help to stretch the hips, glutes, and lower back. Here's how to do it:

Start by sitting on the floor with your legs extended in front of you.

Bend your right knee and place your right foot on the floor in front of you.

Cross your left ankle over your right thigh, so that your left knee is pointing out to the side.

Flex your left foot, pressing your toes toward your left knee.

Use your hands to gently guide your left knee down toward the floor, feeling a stretch in your left hip and glute.

Keep your spine straight and your chest lifted, and breathe deeply in this pose for several breaths.

To come out of the pose, release your left foot and extend both legs in front of you.

Repeat the pose on the other side, crossing your right ankle over your left thigh.

Remember to move slowly and gently during the Figure Four stretch, and to avoid any sudden or jerky movements that could cause injury. If you experience any pain or discomfort, stop immediately and consult a healthcare professional or qualified yoga instructor for guidance. You can also modify the stretch as needed, using props like a block or blanket to help support your body and deepen the stretch.

83

Pigeon pose

The Pigeon pose, also known as the One-Legged King Pigeon Pose or Eka Pada Rajakapotasana, is a yoga posture that can help to stretch the hips, glutes, and lower back. Here's how to do it:

Start on your hands and knees, with your wrists directly under your shoulders and your knees directly under your hips.

Bring your right knee forward and place it on the floor behind your right wrist.

Stretch your left leg out behind you, keeping your toes tucked under and your knee on the floor.

Square your hips as much as possible, with your right hip moving back and your left hip moving forward.

Walk your hands forward, lowering your torso onto your right thigh and extending your arms out in front of you.

Relax your forehead to the floor or onto a block or blanket, if needed.

Breathe deeply in this pose for several breaths, feeling a stretch in your right hip and glute.

To come out of the pose, lift your torso back up and step your right knee back to meet your left knee.

Repeat the pose on the other side, bringing your left knee forward and stretching your right leg out behind you.

Remember to move slowly and gently during the Pigeon pose, and to avoid any sudden or jerky movements that could cause injury. If you experience any pain or discomfort, stop immediately and consult a healthcare professional or qualified yoga instructor for guidance. You can also modify the stretch as needed, using props like a block or blanket to help support your body and deepen the stretch.

Wrist and hand stretches

Working on a computer for extended periods of time can cause tension and stiffness in the wrists and hands. Here are some yoga stretches to help release that tension:

Wrist flexor stretch: Extend your right arm in front of you with your palm facing down. Use your left hand to gently pull your right fingers back toward your wrist until you feel a stretch in your forearm.

Hold for several breaths and then repeat on the other side.

Wrist extensor stretch: Extend your right arm in front of you with your palm facing up. Use your left hand to gently press your right fingers down toward your wrist until you feel a stretch in the back of your forearm. Hold for several breaths and then repeat on the other side.

Prayer hands stretch: Bring your palms together in front of your chest with your fingers pointing up. Slowly lower your hands toward your waist, keeping your palms pressed together and your elbows out to the sides, until you feel a stretch in your wrists and forearms. Hold for several breaths.

Fist stretch: Make a fist with your right hand and then slowly release your fingers, one by one, until your hand is fully extended. Repeat on the other side.

Finger stretch: Place the fingertips of your right hand on a table or other flat surface and gently press down until you feel a stretch in your fingers. Hold for several breaths and then repeat on the other hand.

Remember to move slowly and gently during these stretches, and to avoid any sudden or jerky movements that could cause injury. If you experience any pain or discomfort, stop immediately and consult a healthcare professional or qualified yoga instructor for guidance.

Fist open and close

The fist open and close exercise is a simple yoga stretch that can help to loosen up the fingers, hands, and wrists. Here's how to do it:

Sit comfortably with your back straight and your hands resting on your thighs.

Make a fist with both hands, wrapping your fingers tightly around your thumbs.

Hold the fists for a few seconds, feeling the tension in your fingers and hands.

Slowly release your fingers, one by one, until your hands are fully extended.

Spread your fingers apart as wide as you can, feeling a stretch in your hands and wrists.

Hold the stretch for a few seconds, and then slowly make a fist again.

Repeat the sequence several times, opening and closing your fists at a comfortable pace.

Remember to move slowly and gently during the fist open and close exercise, and to avoid any sudden or jerky movements that could cause injury. If you experience any pain or discomfort, stop immediately and consult a healthcare professional or qualified yoga instructor for guidance.

94

Finger stretch

The finger stretch is a simple yoga exercise that can help to release tension and stiffness in the fingers, hands, and wrists. Here's how to do it:

Sit comfortably with your back straight and your hands resting on your thighs.

Lift your right hand up in front of you, with your palm facing away from your body.

Use your left hand to gently pull each finger of your right hand back towards your wrist, one at a time.

Hold each finger stretch for a few seconds, feeling a gentle stretch in the fingers and hand.

Repeat the stretch on your left hand.

You can also do this stretch with both hands at once by placing the fingertips of each hand together, and then gently pressing your hands together until you feel a stretch in your fingers and hands.

Remember to move slowly and gently during the finger stretch, and to avoid any sudden or jerky movements that could cause injury. If you experience any pain or discomfort, stop immediately and consult a healthcare professional or qualified yoga instructor for guidance.

Yoga routines for office workers

Here are two yoga routines that office workers can use to stretch and relieve tension during the workday:

Quick 5-Minute Routine:

This short routine can be done at your desk or in a small space and can help to relieve tension in the neck, shoulders, back, and wrists.

Begin by taking a deep breath in and raising your arms overhead.

Exhale and release your arms back down to your sides.

Roll your shoulders forward and backward a few times, then shrug your shoulders up to your ears and release them back down.

Gently tilt your head to the right, holding for a few seconds, and then repeat on the left side.

Interlace your fingers behind your back and lift your hands away from your body, feeling a stretch in your chest and shoulders.

Roll your wrists in circles, then switch directions.

Take a few deep breaths, focusing on relaxing any tension in your body.

15-Minute Lunchtime Routine:

This longer routine can be done during your lunch break and includes a variety of stretches to release tension in the neck, shoulders, back, hips, and legs.

Begin in a seated position with your back straight and your feet flat on the ground.

Take a few deep breaths, focusing on relaxing any tension in your body.

Move into a seated forward fold, reaching your hands towards your feet and feeling a stretch in your hamstrings and lower back.

Come up to a standing position and move into a downward-facing dog pose, stretching your arms and legs and feeling a stretch in your shoulders and hamstrings.

From downward-facing dog, move into a low lunge, stretching your hips and legs.

Move into a seated twist, twisting your spine to the right and left.

Finish with a few minutes of relaxation in savasana, lying on your back with your eyes closed and focusing on your breath.

Remember to listen to your body and move slowly and gently during any yoga routine. If you experience any pain or discomfort, stop immediately and consult a healthcare professional or qualified yoga instructor for guidance.

102

Quick morning routine

Here's a quick morning routine that can help to energize your body and prepare you for the day ahead:

Mountain pose: Begin by standing with your feet hip-width apart, arms at your sides, and palms facing forward. Take a few deep breaths and feel the ground beneath your feet.

Forward fold: On your next exhale, bend forward from your hips and let your arms and head hang towards the ground. Relax your neck and shoulders and breathe deeply.

Halfway lift: On your next inhale, lift your torso halfway up and straighten your arms, keeping your back flat and your gaze forward. Downward-facing dog: Step back into downward-facing dog by lifting your hips up and back, and pressing your hands and feet into the ground. Hold for a few breaths and feel the stretch in your hamstrings and calves.

Warrior I: From downward-facing dog, step your right foot forward between your hands and rise up into warrior I pose, with your back foot turned out slightly and your arms raised overhead. Hold for a few breaths and feel the strength in your legs and core.

Chaturanga: Release your arms and step back into plank pose, then lower yourself down to the ground into chaturanga pose. This is a challenging pose, so feel free to modify or skip it if it's too difficult.

Cobra: From chaturanga, press your palms into the ground and lift your chest up into cobra pose, with your elbows bent and your gaze forward.

Child's pose: Release your arms and sit back into child's pose, with your forehead resting on the ground and your arms stretched out in front of you. Take a few deep breaths and feel the stretch in your back and hips.

Repeat on the other side: Step your left foot forward and repeat the sequence from warrior I through child's pose.

This routine should take about 5-10 minutes and can be done anywhere you have space to move. Remember to listen to your body and move slowly and gently, especially if you're new to yoga or have any health concerns.

106

Mid-day routine

Here's a mid-day routine that can help to relieve tension and refresh your body and mind:

Seated spinal twist: Begin by sitting up straight in your chair with your feet flat on the ground. Place your right hand on your left knee and twist your torso to the left, using your left hand to hold the back of your chair. Hold for a few breaths and then switch sides.

Eagle arms: Sit up straight and raise your arms out in front of you at shoulder height. Cross your right arm over your left and wrap your forearms around each other, bringing your palms to touch. Hold for a few breaths and then switch sides.

Seated forward fold: Sit up straight and extend your legs out in front of you. On your next exhale, bend forward from your hips and reach for your toes or ankles. Hold for a few breaths and then release.

Chair pose: Stand up and come to the front of your chair. Bend your knees and lower your hips back as if you were sitting in a chair, and raise your arms overhead. Hold for a few breaths and then release.

Warrior II: Step your left foot back and turn it out slightly, while keeping your right foot pointing forward. Raise your arms out to the sides and gaze over your right fingertips, feeling the stretch in your hips and thighs. Hold for a few breaths and then switch sides.

Tree pose: Stand with your feet hip-width apart and shift your weight onto your left foot. Lift your right foot and place it on your left inner thigh, then press your palms together in front of your chest. Hold for a few breaths and then switch sides.

Savasana: Lie down on your mat or the floor with your arms and legs stretched out, palms facing up. Close your eyes and take a few deep breaths, relaxing your body and mind completely.

This routine should take about 10-15 minutes and can be done in a quiet space or even in your office if you have a private area to practice. Remember to modify or skip any poses that feel uncomfortable or painful, and to take breaks as needed throughout the practice.

End of day routine

Here's an end-of-day yoga routine that can help you unwind and release any stress or tension from your workday:

Child's pose: Begin on your hands and knees, with your big toes touching and your knees hip-width apart. Lower your hips back towards your heels and stretch your arms out in front of you, resting your forehead on the ground. Take a few deep breaths, feeling the stretch in your hips and spine.

Downward dog: From child's pose, lift your hips up and back to come into downward dog. Press your hands and feet into the ground, lengthen your spine, and release any tension in your neck and shoulders. Hold for a few breaths.

Standing forward fold: Step forward to the top of your mat and fold forward from your hips, bringing your hands to the ground or resting them on your shins. Let your head and neck relax and take a few deep breaths.

Low lunge: Step your left foot back and lower your knee to the ground, bringing your hands to your right thigh. Gently press your hips forward, feeling the stretch in your left hip flexor. Hold for a few breaths and then switch sides.

Cobra pose: Lie down on your stomach and place your hands under your shoulders. Press into your hands to lift your chest off the ground, keeping your elbows close to your sides. Hold for a few breaths and then release.

Happy baby pose: Lie on your back and bring your knees towards your chest. Grab the outsides of your feet and gently pull your knees towards the floor, feeling the stretch in your hips and inner thighs.

Seated meditation: Sit cross-legged on your mat or in a chair, with your spine tall and your hands resting on your knees. Close your eyes and take a few deep breaths, letting go of any stress or tension from your day.

This routine should take about 10-15 minutes and can be done in a quiet space at home or in your office. Remember to modify or skip any poses that feel uncomfortable or painful, and to take breaks as needed throughout the practice.

114

Conclusion

In conclusion, practicing yoga stretches can be extremely beneficial for office workers who spend long hours sitting at a desk. Yoga can help improve flexibility, reduce stress and tension, increase energy levels, and improve overall physical and mental health. With the 30 yoga stretches and routines outlined in this book, office workers can easily incorporate yoga into their daily routine and reap the benefits of this ancient practice. Remember to always prioritize safety, listen to your body, and modify or skip any poses that don't feel right for you. With consistent practice, you can improve your physical and mental health, and feel more relaxed and productive throughout your workday.

116

Recap of benefits of yoga stretching for office workers

Here's a recap of the benefits of yoga stretching for office workers:

Improves flexibility and posture

Reduces stress and tension

Increases energy levels and productivity

Boosts mental clarity and focus

Reduces risk of injury and chronic pain

Improves circulation and immune function

Promotes relaxation and better sleep

Enhances overall physical and mental health.

Incorporating yoga stretches into your daily routine can help you feel more comfortable and productive at your desk, while also improving your overall health and wellbeing.

118

Encouragement to incorporate yoga stretching into daily routine

I highly encourage you to incorporate yoga stretching into your daily routine if you're an office worker. The benefits of yoga are numerous and can help improve your physical and mental health, making you feel more comfortable, productive, and energized throughout the day.

Remember that even just a few minutes of yoga stretches can make a big difference in how you feel. You don't need to commit to a long yoga practice to experience the benefits. You can start by incorporating one or two stretches into your routine and gradually build up to a full routine.

Also, don't be discouraged if you don't get the poses right at first. Yoga is a journey, and it takes time and practice to get better. The most important thing is to listen to your body, be patient with yourself, and enjoy the process.

By incorporating yoga stretches into your daily routine, you can improve your physical and mental health, reduce stress, and enhance your overall wellbeing. So, give it a try and see how it makes you feel!

121

Additional resources for further yoga stretching education.

If you're interested in further education on yoga stretching, there are plenty of resources available to help you deepen your practice. Here are a few resources you might find helpful:

Yoga classes: Attending a yoga class can be a great way to learn more about yoga stretching and improve your practice. Look for classes at your local yoga studio or community center.

Online yoga videos: There are many free and paid online yoga videos available that can guide you through a yoga practice. Some popular platforms for online yoga include YouTube, Gaia, and Yoga Journal.

Yoga books: There are countless yoga books available that can help you learn more about the practice, including specific poses and routines. Some popular yoga books include "Light on Yoga" by B.K.S. Iyengar and "The Yoga Bible" by Christina Brown.

Yoga apps: There are many yoga apps available that can guide you through a yoga practice and offer tips and tutorials. Some popular yoga apps include Yoga Studio, Daily Burn, and Glo.

Yoga retreats: If you're looking to deepen your yoga practice, consider attending a yoga retreat. These retreats offer immersive experiences that allow you to focus on your practice and connect with like-minded individuals.

No matter which resource you choose, remember that yoga is a journey, and there is always more to learn. By continuing to educate yourself and deepen your practice, you can experience even more benefits from yoga stretching.

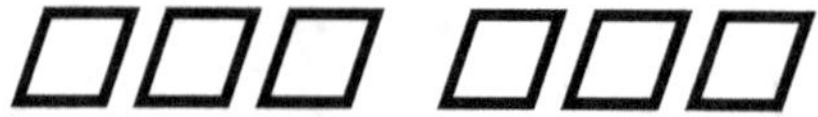